Little Less Dragon Little More Angel

A self help guide to the menopause

Written By

Chris Guyon and Maggie Stanley

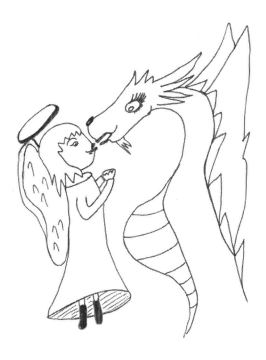

AuthorHouse™ UK Ltd.
500 Avebury Boulevard
Central Milton Keynes, MK9 2BE
www.authorhouse.co.uk
Phone: 08001974150

First published by AuthorHouse 7/24/2009

ISBN: 978-1-4389-9495-6 (sc)

This book is printed on acid-free paper.

Index

Forward

This book came about because Chris Guyon and I are "ladies of a certain age". Before we reached our late 40's we had come across in our work (as therapist and trainers) a number of women struggling with mid life problems, often labelled menopausal or mid life crisis or 'that time of life thingy'!

Clients who were in their middle years were often struggling emotionally and or physically with symptoms put down to that time of life called the menopause. HRT is held up as the wonder treatment to help patients deal with this time of change. Whilst for some women it is a wonder drug, and certainly improves their quality of life, for others it only partially helps or doesn't help at all, or for different reasons they are unable to use the treatment.

We heard clients telling us that they had used a number of approaches to help, such as counselling, prescribed drugs, herbs, oils, as well as some very new age approaches. It started to occur to us that different people had different needs and not everything worked for everyone. The main effects for women were mood swings, fatigue, memory loss/confusion, hot sweat/flushes and irregular, erratic bleeding and loss of confidence.

Then the magic time hit Chris and I, with Chris being peri - menopausal and me menopausal. For me this has been a roller coaster ride of HRT, (which I had to stop on medical grounds), complimentary therapies and various herbs and concoctions, even the menopause cake! I have felt unclean being so hot and sweaty while trying to do my job. I have suffered dehydration on a hot day due to sweating so much. I have forgotten things, lost concentration in the middle of training people and could not remember what I was talking about. I can lose confidence and feel anxious for no reason what so ever. Chris has started to notice things happening to her, mainly erratic menstruation, tiredness and memory failure. At least we laugh about having a brain between us!

The menopause is a natural event in a woman's life so the two of us decided to embark on a journey of discovery to find the best way to negotiate the way through these uncharted waters. There are those few lucky women who have very little problem; however, our experience has been a number of women suffering in silence and in emotional distress which affects their wellbeing. If I am honest this has been the case for me and I wish I had known what I now know. Being cognisant of what to expect, what might happen and ways to help stop or alleviate symptoms can make life so much easier.

I was lucky that having training and a toolbox of techniques at hand I have been able to deal with some of the emotional experiences although it has been hard at times. I did not find information readily available and sadly, although my GP has been as helpful as possible, HRT is all they seem to offer. Chris and I have reflected on our own feelings and symptoms and recognised these in other women so this led us to write this book.

Chris and I are not trying to replace any medical expert or advice. We just want to inform and help women make up their own minds on how to take care of themselves and to navigate the menopause phase in their lives as stress free and comfortable as possible.

If you have any concerns about your health or symptoms we stress the importance of seeing your doctor for a check up.

We surveyed women about the menopause as we wondered what their thoughts were about this time of their life. You can see the results at the back of the book on page 90.

The whole subject of the menopause could be described as the elephant in the room as it is a subject we seem to talk around rather than acknowledge. The poem, The Elephant in the room, by Terry Kettering is talking about a death however it could so easily be talking about the menopause and the way it is avoided.

"We talk about the weather.
We talk about work.
We talk about everything else -
except the elephant in the room."

The Poem was in "Bereavement Magazine" October 1989, Vol 3, No. 8)

However it can be found at the following link -

http://www.compassionatefriendswa.org.au/poetry.htm

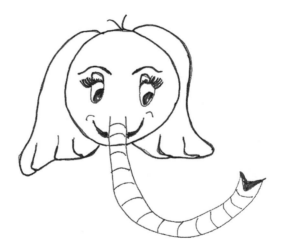

We hope while you read this book that you may laugh a little maybe sigh a little but hopefully find the book a helpful resource that will help you understand the menopause

Maggie Stanley and Chris Guyon

Introduction

Like the song "my favourite things" I can real off the symptoms of the menopause -

> Hot flushing skin, and teenager's spots, flashes of chills and memory lapses, mood swings that frighten and days without sleep; these are a few of my menopausal things.

> When my joints hurt and my head thumps and I'm feeling down I simply remember I'm a menopausal dame and then I don't scream and shout.

It was hard for me to realise I was entering the menopause as I had an early hysterectomy at 37 yrs. I had a remaining ovary that served me well until my mid forties, that is when things started to happen. I was put on HRT at this stage which did help for a time but as soon as I came off my happy patch I shot into the menopause with a vengeance.

I certainly was not prepared for some of the things that happened to my mind and my body. No one ever warned me that having had a hysterectomy that the menopause could be a rougher ride. To think of it, no one ever told me about the menopause, it was that subject women nodded knowingly about but never really talked about.

My mum died in her early fifties and I was the big sister in my family. I had no aunties or older friends who had been through it so I really had no one to ask. It was a case for me to suck it and see and it was a lemon and it was sharp - come to think of it – it was like I had an ulcer in my mouth.

Chris has her own journey that she has started and with our strange sense of humour we are lurching our way through. This is our journey and you are welcome to join us in the places we have visited and the things we have found out. We have laid the book out under specific headings with our input and observations as you go through. You can laugh and cry along with us but all I can say is thank God I had my friend Chris with me because at times I was like a raging teenager. As she said to her daughter when I used a few "f" words to try and explain something "it's ok Cassie Maggie is suffering with menopausal tourettes"

So over to you Chris

Menopause was a word bandied about amongst my friends as we started to hit our 40's. Something you would sometimes laugh about but secretly worry about how it would affect YOU!

Although overweight I was healthy, blood pressure good, no sign of cholesterol problems and a menstrual cycle that was so regular I could almost set my watch by it!

Like Maggie, I didn't really know too much about the mechanics of menopause. I am the eldest of four with three younger brothers, so no big sister to ask. My mother had a total hysterectomy in her early 40's, due to gynae problems, and I had married and left home before her 'forced' menopause kicked in. I DO remember my father making some comments about living "with a mad woman" and my brothers complaining about Mum's unpredictable mood swings. I didn't feel right asking her at the time about menopausal symptoms and as the years went on it never came up in conversation!

When I reached the grand old age of 49 I had started to notice changes in my body and energy levels. My memory also started to let me down – sometimes causing me immense embarrassment! I thought it was 'just one of those things' but then my oh so regular menstrual cycle started to become erratic.

At this point I decided to visit my GP – it was the first time I had met him as I had recently moved to a new area. I explained that I thought I was becoming menopausal and told him what I had noticed changing. He didn't seem very impressed and told me that these symptoms could be caused for other reasons. So, he sent me for blood tests and an MOT with the Practice Nurse.

When I went back for the results he looked at me over the top of his spectacles and said "I'm very happy to say you are still a woman Mrs Guyon, the tests do not show that you are menopausal". I was speechless! (When relaying this event to a group of female GP's at a presentation there was a group gasp of disbelief and one piped up with "and so will you be after I have ripped your testicles off"!!). Of course, my blood tests were not showing high FSH levels because I was Peri-menopausal – the start of the menopause journey.

We would both like to thank the people who have helped us to write this book. The ladies who completed our survey, our husbands, friends who read the book pre publication and Gill who helped to deal with two IT incompetent women.

Chapter 1

Understanding the Menopause

The menopause is a natural event in a woman's life. It could be said that there are three stages to this change in life – peri-menopause, menopause and post menopause. The menopause is a gradual process that happens over time unless surgically or medically induced, such as hysterectomy and chemotherapy. It can be hard not to view the menopause as a natural process given it can give woman symptoms that can cause distress and discomfort. The falling levels of hormones in a woman's bloodstream gives rise to the symptoms that women describe at the time of the menopause. The whole process can take up to 15 years or longer, this period will depend on the partner, the family and other factors.

The things that can happen to your body can be bewildering. Losing your thread of thought, forgetting things, sweating profusely in the middle of winter (and this is natural!) M

"Menopause is defined by the World Health Organization and the Stages of Reproductive Aging Workshop (STRAW) working group: - as the permanent cessation of menstrual periods that occurs naturally or is induced by surgery, chemotherapy, or radiation. Natural menopause is recognized after 12 consecutive months without menstrual periods that are not associated with a physiologic (e.g., lactation) or pathologic cause. Menopausal transition often begins with variations

in length of the menstrual cycle. The hormonal changes during the menopausal transition can span several years."

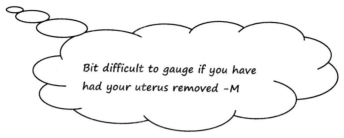

Some women feel a sense of sadness and loss at the time of the menopause; they can also feel a loss of femininity and sexuality. The menopause certainly does not reduce femininity or sexuality and can be viewed as a time of release and freedom and some women revel in the release of the monthly 'curse'.

Research would show that 85% of menopausal women experience some effects from lowering levels of oestrogen with some 25% who actually seek medical intervention.

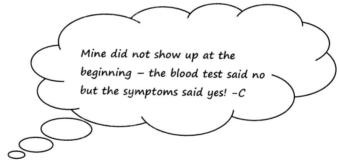

Peri-menopause phase– This is not an officially defined medical term but it is a way to help women to understand how the body is winding down preparing for the menopause. It is referred to as a transition time in some definitions. This process can start at 39-51 years the average time being 45 years. The woman's body begins to produce smaller amounts of the female hormones. Oestrogen and progesterone levels begin to fall and fluctuate with the monthly period becoming erratic and irregular. If a woman is having symptoms she can ask her doctor for a blood test, as it is important to check things out as tests and examination can establish if symptoms are due to the onset of the menopause or other causes.

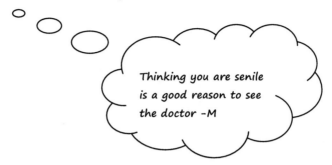

Thinking you are senile is a good reason to see the doctor -M

The Menopause phase– – a natural menopause is when a woman has not had a period for a year, however this can be surgically induced. Although the menopause sees the ceasing of periods it is actually the loss of ovarian function that ends the fertility of a woman. The ovaries cease to produce the levels of oestrogen and progesterone required to maintain the menstrual cycle so the periods stop. This happens when the follicular stimulating hormone fails to activate the ovaries to ovulate. The average age for the menopause is 51 years and it is usual for a daughter to have a menopause at a similar age as her mother. At this time it is important to ensure periods have stopped before contraception is stopped as there is a risk of pregnancy until the periods have ceased for some time.

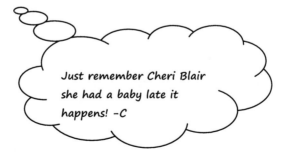

Just remember Cheri Blair she had a baby late it happens! -C

Post menopause phase— this is the time that health related issues can start to appear after the female hormones production has been reduced and egg production has ceased. This is because the protection from the female hormones being produced by the ovaries has been greatly reduced. Chronic conditions may start to appear in women after menopause so it is important that women are aware of some of the potential problems.

- **Cardiovascular disease.** Life style is more important at the time of menopause as heart disease is the leading cause of death in women. There are steps that can be done to reduce the risk of heart disease. These risk-reduction steps are such things as stopping smoking, reducing high blood pressure, taking regular exercise, and eating a healthy diet low in saturated fats and plentiful in whole grains, fruits and vegetables.

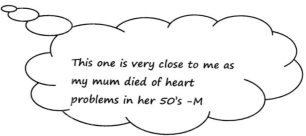

This one is very close to me as my mum died of heart problems in her 50's –M

- **Osteoporosis.** Post menopause there may be a loss in bone density which could increase the risk of osteoporosis which can cause bones to become brittle and weak, leading to an increased risk of fractures. Exercise which include strength training and weight-bearing activities such as walking gardening and jogging are good activities to help maintain bone density and strength.

- **Urinary incontinence.** One of the unfortunate side effects of menopause is that the tissues of the vagina and urethra may lose elasticity. This can result in frequent sudden and strong urges to urinate which can lead to leakage of urine.

- This loss of urine can also occur when coughing, laughing or lifting.

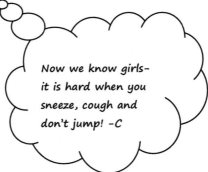

- **Weight gain.** Many women complain about weight gain especially around the stomach region during the menopause. There may be a need to eat fewer calories per day and increase exercise to help maintain weight.

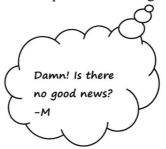

End note - Chris and I wonder how many women out there stress and fret that they are either going mad or are ill when it is just the menopause. Knowledge is so powerful as it puts you in control of your mind and body so that you can then deal with it. It can be for some women that the fear is so great that something is seriously wrong that it creates anxiety about consulting the doctor because of the dread of what might be wrong.

Dr Christiane Northrup in her book Women's Bodies Women's Wisdom says that the menopause is seen in medical circles as a deficiency disease not as a natural process. Women in the menopause are seen as no longer in the child production phase rather in failed production leading to shutdown. This in turn could lead women to think they are shutting down rather that being vital, strong and valuable members of society. This view of how western medicine views the menopause would appear to be upheld by our experiences and of women we have talked to.

You don't see scientists or doctors running around trying to stick falling leaves back on branches during the autumn. This is because it is a natural event so why is it that the menopause is seen as an illness by the medical profession?

It seems to be the luck of the draw if you have a GP who has time to give to patients and not constantly battling against the clock, or better still a GP who has an interest in women's health. The pair of us were invited to give a presentation of our research and workshop to a group of female GP's. They were very interested and admitted they only had eight minutes to talk to their menopausal patients during surgery appointments which are obviously not long enough. Some of the GP's felt that they had learnt something new themselves about the menopause after our presentation.

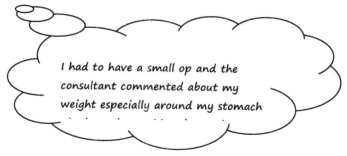

I had to have a small op and the consultant commented about my weight especially around my stomach . . . .

It can help to phone the practice up and ask which doctor specialises in women's health. Someone who specialises will understand symptoms and be able to reassure and suggest the right tests and examinations. Once you know you are OK then you can step forward and embrace the world as the woman you want to be and with out period pains yea!!

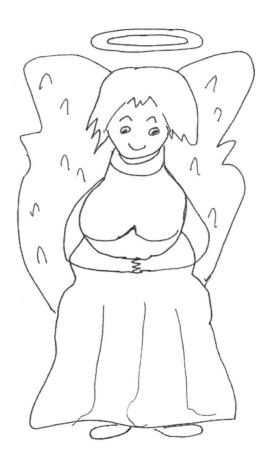

Chapter2

The Symptoms of Menopause

Research would indicate that about 70% of women experience menopausal symptoms. Each woman will experience the menopause in very different ways. Some will have more physical signs and symptoms while some have more emotional and others a combination. There are some women who experience very few symptoms.

Hot Flushes – Changes and fluctuations in oestrogen levels lead to some women experiencing these uncomfortable periods of fluctuating body temperature. No one really understands why they happen, however it is thought that it is due to the autonomic nervous system behaving erratically. This has the effect of causing the blood vessels close to the skin to dilate and trigger the sweat response which happens when an individual gets too hot.

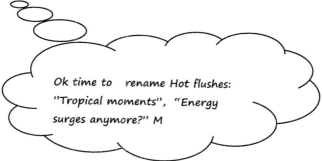

This flushing can happen during the day or night and can lead to disturbed sleep. The menopause affects the temperature control of a woman's body and is connected to blood flow and oestrogen levels in the brain. A hot flush or "tropical moment" usually lasts less than a minute. It is a sudden feeling of heat or warmth spreading over the body sometimes followed by perspiration. The hot flushes will decrease over time and can be an early sign of menopause. Night sweats can be hard to cope with as a woman can wake up drenched in sweat and over-heated only to feel cold a short while later. This night time waking can lead to fatigue during the day and problems waking in the morning.

Mood and memory – Women may experience mood swings, irritability, anxiety and occasional difficulties with memory or concentration. If a woman had the mood swings of the menopause explained to her, that it is similar to going through puberty with raging hormones, it may be easier to understand. Some research would indicate that the changing levels of hormones can trigger the stress response leading to feelings of anxiety, panic, palpitations and memory loss. Often women don't sleep well due to the hot flushes which can also upset mood due to tiredness.

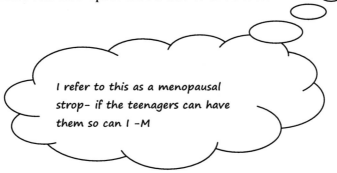

I refer to this as a menopausal strop- if the teenagers can have them so can I -M

Sleep problems – this is discussed under other headings - insomnia can be caused by the night sweats and joint aches and other menopause problems that some women experience.

Bladder problems – During the menopause due to decrease in hormones this can lead to thinning of the tissues lining the bladder and urinary tract, resulting in decreased bladder control or small leaks of urine i.e. when laughing or sneezing. The bladder capacity may be seen to reduce, needing to go to the toilet more frequently.

Susceptibility to urinary tract infections and cystitis may occur at the time or post menopausal.

> My teenage daughter cringed when I started checking out Tena lady in the super market- I prefer sanitary towels any way - C

> Careful girls don't sneeze, cough, laugh or jump with a full bladder or incontinence pants here we come -C

Skin –The skin at the time of the menopause, due to the reduction of oestrogen in the body, can look more wrinkled and aged. This is because oestrogen helps in maintaining collagen within the skin which adds support to the skin. The skin can become itchy and sensitive which is not helped by the hot flushes. As the menopause proceeds and leading on to post menopausal stage the skin may become drier, thinner, less elastic and more prone to bruising.

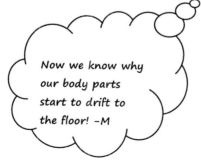

> Now we know why our body parts start to drift to the floor! -M

Hair - women sometimes notice that their hair is not as thick as it used to be, it also has a tendency to be drier. Unwanted growth of hair such as on the face, chest or abdomen can be distressing for some women. This is another side effect of oestrogen reduction.

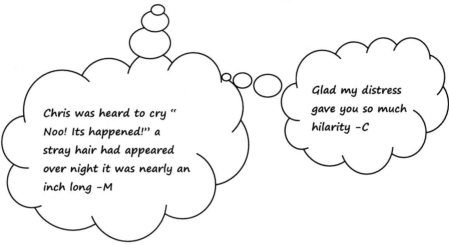

Chris was heard to cry "Noo! Its happened!" a stray hair had appeared over night it was nearly an inch long -M

Glad my distress gave you so much hilarity -C

Sexual factors –Reduction of oestrogen may cause vaginal dryness and skin thinning, which can result in painful intercourse and a possibility of infections. The lowered hormone levels can also affect the blood flow to the sexual organs and libido may be reduced. This is discussed later in the book.

Vaginal bleeding/menstruation –This appears to vary woman to woman, some bleed irregularly with no periods for a couple of months whilst others may have unpredictable excessive bleeding. This is due to the falling off of ovulation due to decrease in fertility. Women need to take care of falling pregnant whilst having irregular periods and check out irregular bleeding as it can be caused by fibroids or other gynealogical problems.

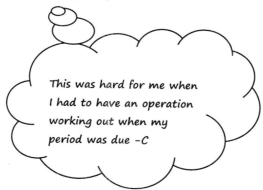

This was hard for me when I had to have an operation working out when my period was due -C

Joint aches – An increase in joint aches and back aches can be as a result of the decrease in oestrogen.

Heart Palpitations during the menopause are thought to be caused by fluctuating hormones such as oestrogen and progesterone. These usually go away as the hormones begin to settle down and level out. It is important to get the palpations checked out as it could indicate other underlying conditions.

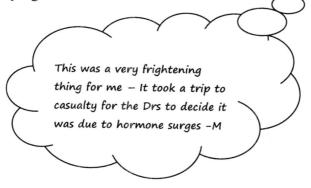

This was a very frightening thing for me – It took a trip to casualty for the Drs to decide it was due to hormone surges -M

Body shape -The body stores fat in different places during the fertile years. It collects on the hips and thighs and bottom. At the menopause it gets laid down as abdominal fat. During the menopause muscle mass declines which results in a fall in the Basal Metabolic

Rate. The body has less of the energy burning areas so even if calorie input has not increased or diet is unchanged weight can be gained.

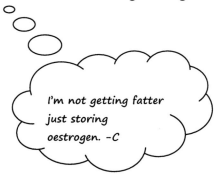

End note- Tammy Wynette wrote the lyric "sometimes it's hard to be a woman" and I think this is true. I certainly found some of the physical changes I have experienced so far have caused me to worry. It was not until we started writing this book that I talked to Chris about some of the fears I had faced. The worst one for me was the worry eating away in my mind that I had early dementia. I was forgetting things; I could not think of words. This meant that objects, places and people became that thing. This could be frustrating not to mention embarrassing when trying to deliver training and I am struggling to think of a word.

I love the following explanation from Chris which made me feel a whole lot better not to mention relieved. So over to Chris -

Whilst researching memory loss linked with menopause I came across an explanation that literally had me laughing out loud! Apparently, when of child-bearing age our memory is focused on keeping our off-spring safe, so if your child was in danger you could react quickly e.g.

"Hey, Johnny, get off that rock, there's a snake coming"

Fast forward 30 or so years and hormone levels fluctuating because now no longer of child-bearing age and the above becomes

"Hey, watchamacallit, get off that bumpy thing, there's a thingammy coming"

Not quite the same impact!

But now we know WHY this happens it makes it a whole lot easier to understand and cope with these 'menopausal moments' as Maggie and I like to call them.

One lady I know calls these CRAFT moments. The polite version is

"Can't Remember Any Flipping Thing"

Another bit of advice for when people ask "how are you?" When you say "fine" be careful as you are telling them that you are

F**d Up**

Insecure

Neurotic and

Emotional

Come to think of it when you are feeling menopausal and you say "fine" the interpretation above could be really how you are feeling. On a serious note how often do you say you are fine and the reality is that you are not?

Chris and I do try not to say fine. If we do and slip and say the offending word there is a raise of an eyebrow and the word repeated back FINE?

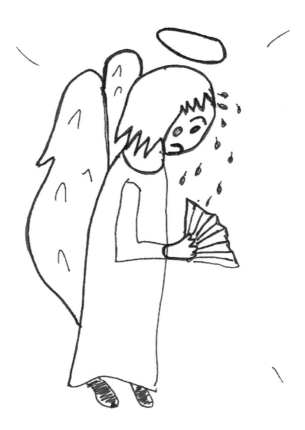

Chapter3

A problem or Metamorphosis - The emotional side of the menopause

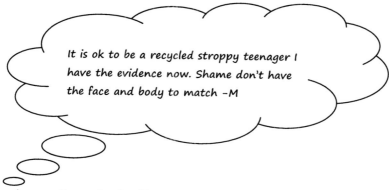

It is ok to be a recycled stroppy teenager I have the evidence now. Shame don't have the face and body to match -M

The change from the fertile years to the non-fertile years can be viewed like puberty. When the hormones rise the body has to cope with the changes, which can put a strain on the individual physically and mentally. Not every woman goes through the mood swings during menopause some sail through with an air of serenity.

Mood swings do vary from tearfulness to depression and does not last long with some but can be difficult for others. Looking at the research there is some evidence that the chemical changes due to the menopause can cause emotional and behavioural upsets. However, researching this area appears to have been a difficult one as emotional upsets can be caused for many different reasons and it is hard to pinpoint the menopause as the cause. There is a theory that links low mood with fluctuating hormone levels due to the menopause, resulting in periods of sadness, hopelessness with some experiencing depression.

Anecdotally talking to women who are menopausal

with emotional aspects that have come about since entering the menopausal stage of their life.

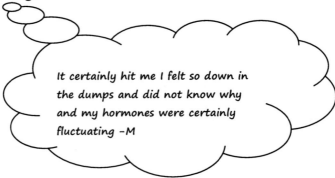

It certainly hit me I felt so down in the dumps and did not know why and my hormones were certainly fluctuating -M

The physical side of the change of life such as hot flushes, memory loss, fatigue, pain and dry vagina can have an impact on how a woman feels and behaves. Feeling hot and sweaty and losing sleep or feeling an idiot for not being able to remember things can soon erode self confidence. A hot flush can mimic an anxiety or panic attack or forgetting things can be a frightening experience especially for a normally confident and capable woman.

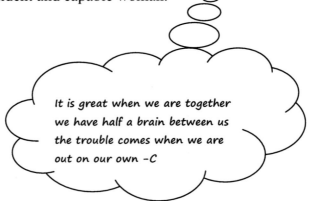

It is great when we are together we have half a brain between us the trouble comes when we are out on our own -C

When these chemical changes begin to occur within a woman there is an awareness of starting to age. In this media driven time of youth, feeling you are getting old can lead to feeling of loss, of being no use and past your sell by date. It is possible that a spouse or partner is facing similar feelings of aging, often called the mid life crisis.

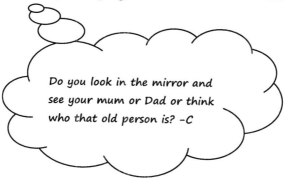

Do you look in the mirror and see your mum or Dad or think who that old person is? -C

There are many facts and reasons within a woman's life around the time of the menopause, despite the chemical changes within her body that could result in her emotional stability and well being affected. Women often become labelled unfairly at this time for being an emotional volcano but they are often dealing with everyone else's emotional baggage, and find it hard to say **enough!**

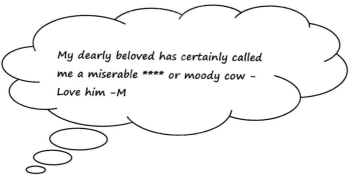

My dearly beloved has certainly called me a miserable **** or moody cow – Love him -M

The hormone levels and changes within the body at this time can cause mood swings which lead to increasing irritability and low mood which makes life difficult. If the individual is depressed or anxious there will be other factors that will have increased the likelihood of clinical depression and anxiety. Previous episodes of depression, life events, personality, levels of support, ability to managing stress, attitude and belief systems will all have an effect that can lead to deterioration of mental health. An individual's internal world and what is going on in their life can combine with the bodily changes to create a change in mental wellbeing.

Who is going to miss period pains? -C

Such aspects can be-

- **Ageing** -a woman may feel negative about growing older and that the menopause is a stage that is to be dreaded and feared. Negative thinking and mental attitude can lead to an increase in symptoms so coping mechanisms are an important factor with mental wellbeing at this time for a woman.

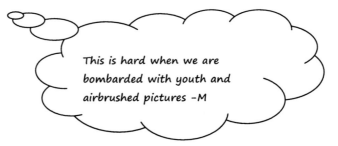

This is hard when we are bombarded with youth and airbrushed pictures -M

- **Role** –In this period of time in a woman's life a number of changes can be taking place and the feeling of being needed and having value may be diminishing. At work there may be nowhere to go on the promotion front or career development or nearing retirement. Children leaving home, going to Uni, setting up home with a partner or just growing up and not needing so much help. It can also be a time of having too many roles supporting the family, work and becoming a carer for either parents or grandchildren.

On the positive side this time of life can be seen as an opportunity for women to change career and see this stage as an opportunity to have more time and begin to pursue their own interests.

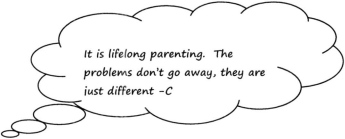

I must confess I am looking forward to this part I feel I have done my bit for society now it is my turn -C

- **Relationships** – relationships are very important. The calibre of the relationship can have an impact on menopause symptoms. Women who are widowed, divorced or separated do tend to suffer more with depressive illness regardless of the fact that they are going through the menopause. If a relationship is not a nurturing and caring one when a woman is menopausal it could be a time when flaws become magnified. The menopause can be blamed for many things and it could be a woman become less tolerant at the time of the menopause

It is lifelong parenting. The problems don't go away, they are just different -C

- **Children** – The menopause is when women become aware *that the reproductive time of their life is coming to an end.* For some women this is a positive thing no more periods and an end to contraception. For other women it can be very hard to face an end of their fertility. In society today with women having children later in life the looming menopause could be something to fear and dread.

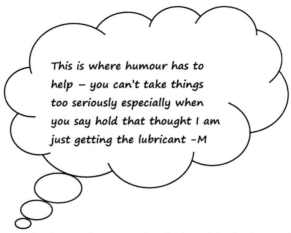

This is where humour has to help – you can't take things too seriously especially when you say hold that thought I am just getting the lubricant -M

- **Sexuality** – desire and a sexual relationship is dependant *on a number of factors not just hormones and the menopause.* The quality of the relationship, self worth, body image, confidence, health and state of mind can affect libido and desire. Sex may have been a little painful and fear and tension can make it difficult on subsequent occasions. An understanding partner and finding ways around aspects of the menopause and aging can be overcome successfully. It is the stress, fear and anxiety that can cause problems on both sides. It is important to remember men have sexual problems too and also can go through a decrease in sexual hormones which can affect the sexual relationship with their partner.

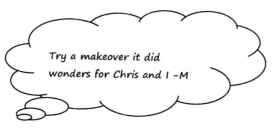

Try a makeover it did
wonders for Chris and I -M

- **Body Image** – Women are more likely to put weight on at this time and if they have always struggled with weight having the issue increase can be enough to lower mood and self worth. It could be that a woman has never had problems and suddenly they begin to put weight on. This can lead to feelings of being a failure especially if they have always had control over their weight. Hair and skin can also change hair can thin and skin be more fragile so it is trying to learn how to deal with the change. Women become more sensitive and view every blemish and line with dread and negativity.

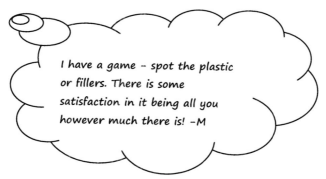

I have a game – spot the plastic
or fillers. There is some
satisfaction in it being all you
however much there is! -M

- **Cultural and Social Influences** – How a culture views a menopausal woman can affect their view of their worth. In some cultures it is a time to be revered and respected by the community. In Western society, where youth is so highly prized, it can lead to feelings of lack of self worth, value and dissatisfaction with being a beautiful older women who has experience and charm.

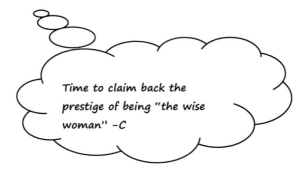

Time to claim back the prestige of being "the wise woman" -C

- **Support** – Especially at this time supportive friendships are important. Depression is less likely to set in when things can be discussed and normalised. The release valve of being able to tell someone how you are feeling and thinking. It can be frightening to have emotions and moods swinging especially if you are a person who is usually in control. Looking after mental wellbeing is important at any stage of life; however it would appear that some women become more vulnerable at the time of the menopause, whether it is due to physical, mental or spiritual things or a combination of all aspects. Women are not always good at looking after themselves. They prioritise others and it is not a priority to look after their own well being at this time. Coping with emotions at any time of life is not always easy; it can be difficult when women who are usually very good at coping and caring for others need to take time out to care for themselves. The menopause unfortunately comes at a time in life when many things are happening for others within the family, work and support network. The woman puts feelings and self care aside often until they become such a problem that they need to be addressed. If action is not taken and feelings and emotions not addressed this can lead to stress, depression, anxiety and panic attacks.

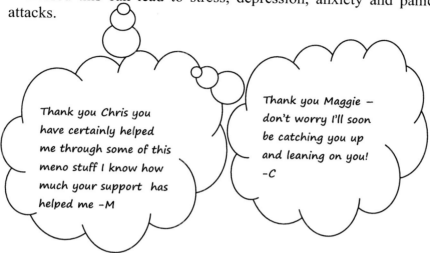

Thank you Chris you have certainly helped me through some of this meno stuff I know how much your support has helped me -M

Thank you Maggie – don't worry I'll soon be catching you up and leaning on you! -C

Depression - It is thought that the menopause can trigger periods of depression in some women. Research would indicate that between 8% and 15% of women in the menopause experience depression. Depression seems likely to hit during peri-menopause, leading up to menopause. One theory, as already suggested above is that the stress of menopause symptoms leads to stress and depression. Woman find symptoms of menopause are simply too difficult to manage with all the other pressures and demands they have on a day to day basis. It can just be the final thing that tips them from coping to not coping.

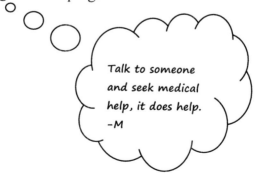

Talk to someone and seek medical help, it does help. -M

A woman is likely to experience depression during menopause if there is a history of depression, anxiety and panic disorders in particular if this happened in their 20s. Women who have had to undergo a hysterectomy and therefore have a surgically induced menopause have an increased risk for depression. Again it needs to be stressed that mid life can be a stressful time for a number of reasons or a time of big changes, so it is not all about the menopause.

If your mood is so low and you feel out of control or unable to cope or have suicidal thoughts it is vital to visit your doctor as soon as possible. There is life after the menopause and life and self management can play a big part in helping to go through this stage of life

End Note It is easy to fall into the low mood state, for some women this is something that they endure silently during the menopause. Chris and I have certainly found this with some women in the courses that we run. They are so relieved to find others feel and think as they do.

I can say this part of the menopause has affected me. I have suffered from low mood and sudden lack of confidence. I am usually out going and full of beans but in the last few years some days it has been a struggle which has frightened and concerned me. I think that the hot flushes and disturbed sleep have added to the low mood. There were days where I could not be bothered. I think people who know me would say that motivation is not one of my weaknesses, however this moodiness I can drop into can pull you down and de-motivate you and don't know why.

Chris and a few of my close friends have been a great help to me. I could be silly or stupid and they would listen and not tell me to pull myself together but empathise and help me through these feelings. In some ways it was like this confusion and lack of confidence was the same as you have when going through puberty. When Chris and I researched the menopause it was great to begin to understand the journey events and rock blocks that I was experiencing with the menopause.

One thing that Chris and I have noticed is that we actually are not so nurturing. This has been a slow change however we have found that suddenly you notice that you have changed. It can creep up on you and if not careful you can begin to worry why this is.

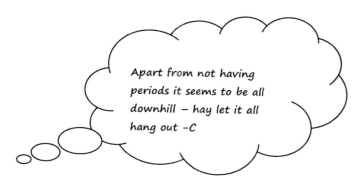

Apart from not having periods it seems to be all downhill – hay let it all hang out -C

The two of us were talking the other day about our husbands and how they have enjoyed their backs being massaged or stroked especially after a hard day. In the last few years instead of just being our nurturing selves we remarked how we started saying "what about my back I have had a hard day too?" This has been a change in our behaviour. We giggled at the thought of the husband's bottom lip protruding and the way they look very bewildered as to why their backs are not so easily massaged as before.

We have noticed that other women say that they used to be so caring and nurturing and now they are not as they use to be. Well girls there is a reason for it, yes you have guessed it is the hormones. As we get older and the hormones diminish this is why hubby's back rub is not so forth coming. When I told my dearly beloved I think his answer was something like "Oh so that explains it" the bottom lip still protruded and he entered his cave. Wait till we write the book on the male menopause!

Maybe this is why in some cultures the older women are known as the wise women as they are less focussed on the nurturing and can see things from a different perspective. Post menopause a woman's bodily energy is focused on other functions not any longer on fertility and reproduction. Well it is just a thought.

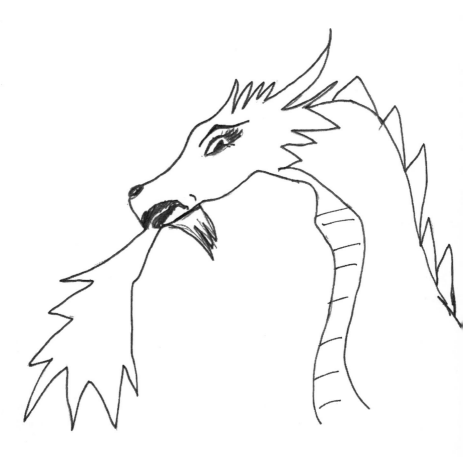

Chapter 4

Sexual life and the menopausal woman

The sexual side of life does not have to come to an end just because a woman is menopausal or post menopausal. Woman at this time of life can and do enjoy a fulfilling sex life. Some women do experience painful or uncomfortable love making but things can be done to alleviate or reduce this side effect of the menopause. As has been explained in other parts of this self help book, when the ovaries decline in activity the oestrogen levels fall in the body causing vaginal changes which can lead to the skin thinning, vaginal dryness due to lack of lubrication and decrease in blood flow to the pelvic area.

Yup this happened to me. It was on researching this book that I realised what was wrong -M

This problem can be extremely distressing and embarrassing. Research seems to differ as to how wide spread the problem is. Some research indicate that 1 in 3 women and some say up to 50% of women experience this problem during and after the menopause. However not many appreciate things can be done to help this upsetting problem. It is often when a woman has problems such as vaginal dryness that she suffers in silence and tries to avoid sexual contact with her partner. This in turn can have a knock on effect within the relationship as the partner can feel hurt and rejected.

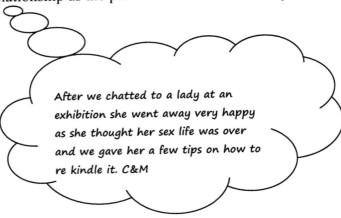

After we chatted to a lady at an
exhibition she went away very happy
as she thought her sex life was over
and we gave her a few tips on how to
re kindle it. C&M

The solution falls into different categories
- **Local oestrogen therapy** - These are inserted into the vagina to help restore the tissue and ease the pain of intercourse. They are inserted 2-3 times per week and help to avoid symptoms. They do not have to be used inserted prior to intercourse. These products come in two basic types
  - Vaginal pesserries
  - Vaginal rings
- **Hormone replacement therapy (HRT)** - This drug option helps to alleviate oestrogen deficiency symptoms. HRT can help local vaginal problems, however these products do not always deal with the problem and sometimes women may have to use local products as well
  - Skin patch usually places on the thigh and are in situ for a few days
  - Oral tablet taken by mouth daily
- **Lubricants** - Some women are not suited to the above products or do not wish to take them. It could be that the problem is not that severe and would prefer to use a lubricant. These products need to be applied each time prior to intercourse and can be a bit inconvenient. There are a number

of products available and a trip to the local pharmacist will offer a number of products. The most widely known product available is KY jelly; however there are a number on the market now. KY jelly is water soluble and may not offer the lubrication required so it is important to seek help and advice. Avoidance of soap may help in the vaginal area and replacing with water based cream to cleanse this area. A vaginal moistening cream/gel may aid this problem seek health professional or pharmacist help to recommend products.

It is important that a woman talks to a health care professional such as a practice nurse or a GP as they will be able to advise and guide them through the different options. They are fully aware that some women do not want to use hormone replacement therapy and will advise on the best products available that have the evidence to back them up. It is not always easy to bring the subject up about vaginal and sexual problems. Some women find that talking to a female health professional easier than a male. When making an appointment to see a doctor or nurse at the surgery ask to see a female rather than a male. Make a list of what the problems are and try to think about how bad or difficult the particular problem is. When we are anxious or embarrassed it is easy to forget things. Be as open and honest as possible, often things that we don't think are important can be significant and help in diagnosis.

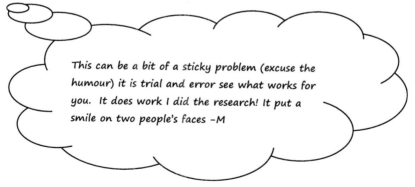

This can be a bit of a sticky problem (excuse the humour) it is trial and error see what works for you. It does work I did the research! It put a smile on two people's faces -M

A number of pharmacists have a consultation room or private area and if you are embarrassed or just don't want to ask for help publicly it may be possible to talk privately. Pharmacists have a lot of knowledge about products and are trained to offer help.

It is not just vaginal problems that can cause problems, it can also be other aspects of the menopause such as

- Hot flushes, not wanting someone up close and personal when you are already overheating.

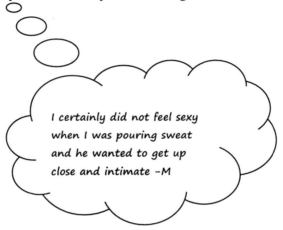

I certainly did not feel sexy when I was pouring sweat and he wanted to get up close and intimate –M

- Some women simply lose the desire to make love as explained in other parts of this book this can be for a variety of different reasons.

  o Loss of hormone

  o Loss of confidence

  o Body Image

- Hot flushes

- Pain and discomfort

- Life stage complications

- Depression/stress

- Stress urinary incontinence

- Weight gain

- Insomnia

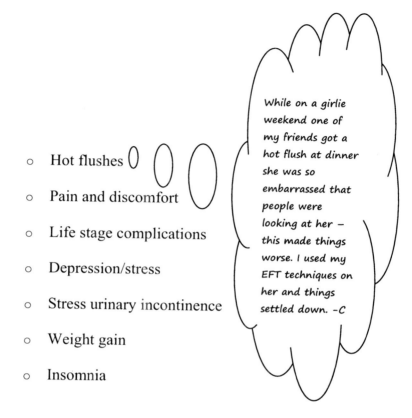

While on a girlie weekend one of my friends got a hot flush at dinner she was so embarrassed that people were looking at her – this made things worse. I used my EFT techniques on her and things settled down. –C

End Note

Communication is important; so many women do not talk to their partners about what is happening to their bodies. Things are often put down to being moody or menopausal. The trouble is as we get older sometimes things have to change. It may be that the way making love has happened before may have to change slightly. In a loving and caring relationship this should be something that can be discussed and ways found to overcome the initial problems. The difficulties may not be entirely due to the woman, the partner may be having a few difficulties too. If a discussion can take place between the couple then it could be that both partners may need to seek help from their GP to see what support they can access.

It is not all doom and gloom, for some women their sexual life dramatically improves after menopause and they have an enjoyable and active sex life. Maintaining a close relationship is important with the partners in our lives who can find this time confusing and hurtful.

In this stage in a couple's life penetrative sex can become less important. Instead go back to when you first started dating. Become inventive on doing things rather than going all the way. Arousal can still happen and it helps to take the pressure off either partner to "perform". This approach can help a partner who may be having erectile problems. Learning to enjoy sensual touch can certainly help to keep a relationship intimate.

This intimacy in my relationship is important and one that was slipping away due to plumbing problems, lack of lubrication and overheating. To be honest I think fear played a part, over time I had not realised that the menopause was having on me. I did not want making love to hurt or be sore. The remedy was one I could bring about and once I recognised what the problems was I could deal with it.

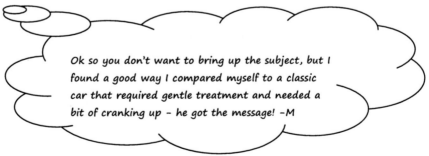

Ok so you don't want to bring up the subject, but I found a good way I compared myself to a classic car that required gentle treatment and needed a bit of cranking up - he got the message! –M

We have certainly had a few giggles and fun on the way. Life does not have to be upsetting and serious, imagination and explaining things in a way your partner can understand is important. I think I used an analogy of a classic car and an electronic circuit diagram he got the message.

It is so easy to let things go and allow thoughts creep in that things are at an end. It is good to wind my daughter up and see the horror in her eyes that her mum may still have an active sex life. I made certain I did not let it go. I still get headaches ladies he can't have it all his way! Maggie

When Maggie use to e-mail me sections of the book for editing my 18 year old daughter would refuse to read out anything from this section of the book. This was because in her words "You don't need to know this Mum you're too old!" Chris

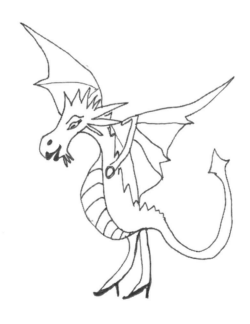

Chapter5

Managing the menopause

There are things that can be done to help women in the short term to alleviate menopausal symptoms; however, some symptoms require more attention and in some cases life style and life choices have to be addressed. Today it is often the case that people are told what to do to improve health and life choices in the media and via the NHS. If individuals are given a reason for adopting a change in life style which will help or alleviate symptoms, and one which has benefits, then it is more likely that a change will be made.

There are many remedies and advice over the years that have been suggested, recommended and advocated to help with and alleviate the symptoms and side effects of the menopause. There has been research into the effectiveness of some products and remedies which do not always come out as effective treatments. Anecdotally some women swear by particular approaches or remedies, while others remain ambivalent or refute effectiveness.

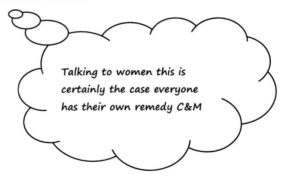

Talking to women this is certainly the case everyone has their own remedy C&M

Approaches for managing the menopause range from self help strategies, medical intervention, complimentary medicine, psychological approaches, herbal remedies and the more wacky and off the wall methods. It would appear that when women are given the opportunity to explore the options and understand the process of change during the menopause, they can decide the ideal option for their lives and body.

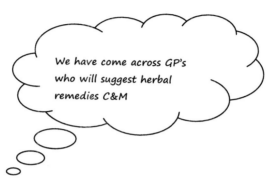

We have come across GP's who will suggest herbal remedies C&M

Most general practitioners in the last few years have become more informed about the menopause and how it can affect a woman's life. Many women "suffer" in silence with menopausal symptoms and are most likely go to the doctor only when things become unbearable. Some doctors will offer advice about alternative treatments such as soy products or black cohosh. The NHS is an evidence based service so a health professional will look at the evidence base and quality of the research to support a remedy, advice or recommendation and give their opinion accordingly.

Not every woman is able to, or wants to take hormone replacement therapy (HRT). Some women thrive on HRT while others have problems and are unable to continue. For those who neither wish to take HRT or are unable to do so often explore different approaches to deal with menopausal symptoms. Women know their own bodies and are the best people, to decide what is the appropriate way to help them negotiate the menopause.

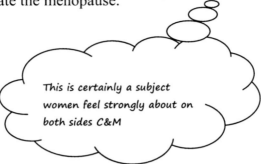

This is certainly a subject women feel strongly about on both sides C&M

End note

Chris has only just started the menopause journey and is just beginning to look at aids and strategies to help her. I have been on this journey for a few years now. The thing that I have found most difficult was coming on and off HRT. I was advised by my GP at 47 years of age that HRT would be helpful for some of the symptoms I was having. What surprised me, and I have heard this from other women, is that I started the menopause all over again when I stopped using HRT. The reason I stopped the first time was that I was fed up with the eczema I developed on my thigh from the patch. Having stopped I found that I did not like the symptoms and I felt very down so I was advised to start again.

After a year of use my blood pressure went up and so I had to stop. This second time I came off HRT the menopause symptoms were worse. I am not saying it would be the case for all women; however it was certainly the case for me. The thing I found most difficult when I first stopped taking HRT was the emotional roller coaster I found myself on and if I am honest I felt very down on a few occasions. This was a strange experience as I knew in one part of my head I was ok but in the other it was like an alien flood of emotions that did not feel my own. It was quite scary at times because this was not me and when I did the research into HRT I realised that I was having menopause symptoms again.

When my dear elderly dogs died within four weeks of each other I was obviously very upset. However I found my emotions all over the place. What I am trying to explain is normally I do my crying and grieving in private. I have faced many things in the past and how I hate to cry in front of people. This time I was bursting into tears and could not talk about my "boys" without sobbing in front of people, some who I hardly knew, which was embarrassing. My emotions were so heightened that the slightest thing would start me off. This was certainly not me and felt like I was premenstrual most of the time.

The things I found helpful at this time were Star Flower Oil, St John's Wort (caution here please check with your pharmacist before taking as it can interact with other drugs), Reiki, EFT and challenging thinking errors. A good soak in the tub with a drop of lavender oil and meditation music is a great tonic.

One thing that certainly helps to lift the spirits is a good blub with a mate who allows you to ramble emotionally (Chris certainly had a soggy shoulder at this time). A few glasses of wine are great, the trouble is it does not help the hot flushes the sacrifices we make!

Kathleen Griffin In her book After the Change says that every woman has her own menopause and experiences it in her own way. She also found during her research how positive women were when they had passed through the menopause. She poses the suggestion that the post menopause woman "is no longer prey to overwhelming forces, she is herself and she and her body are one". I wait with baited breath when I can feel like this most of the time, not oasis in between menopausal moments.

In the next section of the book we have tried to give the reader a wide choice to help the menopause.

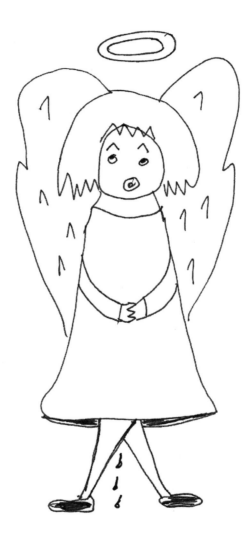

Chapter 6

Self Help Section

Support and help can be resourced from many areas. It is important when choosing a therapist that they are insured and belong to an association and abide by a code of ethics.

Below are some suggestions that may be helpful. We are not recommending any in particular, however we are able to tell you the ones we have tried or have knowledge of.

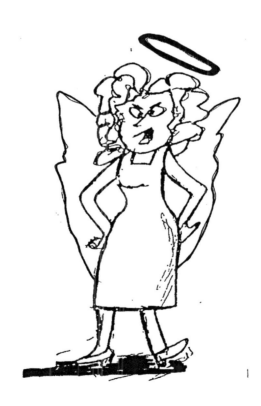

Suggestion	Information	Comments from Chris and Maggie
	Practical help/products	
Advice websites/Self help books	Some are good some are medical based and some are very New Age. At the back of the book are the ones we have found most helpful.	We have found some very good sites and books but some have not been so helpful. The sites from the USA Canada and Aus seem to be good. Books we have found helpful are in the index at the back.
Aromatherapy oils	Aroma therapists can give a massage using specific oils that can help with menopausal symptoms. They can also give you a mixture of oils to use away from treatments. Aroma therapists are trained to know about oils and how to mix them.	Women have told us that aroma therapy has been very good. We have found geranium and lavender oils to be good. Maggie and I have used oils and think they can be a great help. Some oils have a caution about their use so it is important to talk to someone who knows about oils.
Australian Flower remedies/ Bach Flower remedies	Flower essences are very good to help with anxiety and the more emotional side of the menopause. Some flower essences do specific mixtures for menopause. Rescue Remedy can be very good for anxiety or panics.	Olive is good if you are mentally tired. There are such things as Women's Essence and Menopausal Essences that you will find in Health Shops. Maggie and I have used Olive and Rescue Remedy and think they are great. Have used the special essences and not found them any good

Bedding/Clothing	There are companies that make bedding and clothes for women who are having night sweats. However keeping to more natural fibres such as cotton and avoiding synthetic fabrics can help as the natural fibres are more absorbent.	Stretchy synthetic tops are not the right thing for hot flushes. Good old fashioned cotton or linen are good. Cotton night wear does help and avoiding too much poly-cotton in the sheet can help on those hot sweaty nights. Shame about the ironing.-M
Chillo Pillow	This is filled with cold water is like a sponge inside and helps the body to cool down when having night sweats.	Although this is a strange thing, when night sweats are in full flow this little pillow does help, although not everyone's cup of tea, it certainly helped me –M
Diet	Diet can vary from avoiding tea/coffee and spicy food to a more involved plan of eating to ensure good mineral vitamin and hormone making foods.	Diet is very personal it is trial and error. Some things do help like cutting down on caffeine and alcohol, especially if you are in the middle of hot flushes. Diet can make a big difference. Refer to the section on diet.
Exercise	Any exercise is better than none at all it needs to be enjoyable and an activity that will be maintained. This can come in any form walking, exercise class, dance, the gym, sports tuition, sport, gardening.	The key to exercise is fun and if it is enjoyable it will be sustainable. In some ways activity that gets the heart beating and load bearing exercise. The two of us have had fun talking about different forms of load bearing activities and we are not talking about the gym. We do talk about this topic more in depth in the previous sections.

Herbal remedies	There is some evidence base to back these remedies up and some women will swear by these remedies. There are qualified herbalists who can make up tinctures and teas. Most health shops have staff trained to give some guide to products.	I have found sage tincture good for hot flushes but sadly other products not so good. I like things to work quickly and some things you have to take for several weeks. A note of caution these herbal remedies can interact with prescription and other drugs so it is important to check preferable with a health professional if in doubt.-M
Homeopathic remedies	These can be bought over the counter; however a qualified homeopath will work out the best remedy and strength for life style and personality.	In the early days of the menopause I used a homeopath who was able to give me homeopathic remedies which certainly helped me.- M
Make over help	Some makeup artists will come to the home like party plan. Most big stores will do makeup make overs. Skin tones change and make up can look dated. Some organisations run courses in makeup and colour such as Colour Me Beautiful.	Both of us have had make overs and what a difference, it certainly helps to boost self confidence. C& M
	Classes	
Local clubs, activities and voluntary work	Having an interest and becoming involved in local clubs and organisations can help to lift mood. This type of activity can be helpful where there are feelings of loneliness or	Watch point it is easy to take on too much and become over burdened so it is important to say no. We have both been there. – C

	empty nest syndrome	
Meditation classes	Not everyone knows how to relax and turn the chatter in the brain off. Learning to meditate for some is a good way to relax and let the body be peaceful and calm	Both Maggie and I use meditation and believe it is important. It certainly helps to calm things down and can help to bring down a hot flush. –C
Tai Chi Classes/ Yoga Classes	Either of these activities can help to reduce stress as well as increase strength and flexibility. They are not rushing around activities but calm and measured.	I find these activities a bit slow for me however Chris has done Tai Chi and rates that highly. Tai Chi is now taught in the NHS as a stress reliever. – M
	Complimentary therapy and treatments	
Acupuncture	Uses small needles at various points on the body to help with many different problems.	The idea of sticking tiny needles in does not appeal to everyone. However it helped me when I hurt my neck, it relieved the pain.
Aromatherapy	Use of massage and oils to alleviate stress and physical and emotional problems	We talked about the use of oils previously.
Colour	balances and enhance the body's energy which helps	The colours you wear and the colour of your home can affect

therapy	to stimulate the body's own healing	you. If you are suffering from hot flushes wearing red clothing or having red walls in your bedroom may not help. C& M
Crystal therapy	Working with crystal energy can help the body to find its natural rhythm	Chris and I hold our citrine and blue lace crystals close to us as they help with the menopause. M
EFT	It is an emotional version of acupuncture, with no needles. Tapping with the finger tips is used to stimulate well established energy points	Both Maggie and I are EFT practitioners and swear by the technique. It is good for both physical and emotional aspects of the menopause (see EFT for hot flushes) .- C
Indian Head Massage	The massage focuses mainly on the head neck and shoulders. It helps to relax tense areas and rebalance the body.	I am a IHM practitioner and find it really helps to relax people. It is also a massage that can be done seated and required very little clothing to be removed.- M
Massage	Massage is a very powerful form of therapy. Some people love the therapy whilst others hate the idea of being touched. For those who find it hard to relax any form of massage can help to relax the body both physically and mentally.	We both like massage but don't touch Chris's feet. M

Shiatsu	Shiatsu is done fully clothed and involves pressing points and massage on the body. It is said to release energy blocks in the body. Shiatsu uses some of the same point and techniques as acupressure and acupuncture without the needles.	I have had a few treatments which I found good although I think I prefer an aromatherapy massage. C
Reflexology	This therapy massages the feet. Reflexology works on the principal that each part of the foot is linked to a part of the body. The technique applies pressure to certain parts of the foot to bring about relaxation and healing in the body.	As Chris can't stand her feet being touched it is up to me to talk about this. I think this therapy is great I have had it several time and have been very impressed. I have always been amazed at what they can tell from your feet.-M
Reiki	An ancient form of healing that can be done either hands on or off. There is no massage involved and everyone stays fully dressed. It can be done either lying down or sitting in a comfortable chair. The Reiki practitioner is a channel for this high vibrational energy and accesses this energy through the crown of the head and out through the palms of the hands into the energy system of the	We are both Reiki Masters and have been practising for 11yrs (in fact that is how we first met!). We have both found this to be a wonderful method of relaxation and balancing our energies.-C

	person receiving. It works on many levels, physical/emotional/mental and spiritual	
	Emotional/ psychological	
Anger Management/ Anxiety Management/ Assertive training /Depression management/ Stress management training	These four types of psycho/ social courses can be very beneficial sometimes. Learning to deal with ourselves and how to have coping strategies can save hours of counselling. Attending a course that helps to recognise behaviours and then find ways of managing can be extremely empowering for an individual.	Although I teach these types of course I had to first learn and recognise my behaviour for me to learn good assertive skills. Understanding thinking errors certainly helped to de stress my life. M
Counselling	There are many different types of counselling. It is not a failure to feel you need this type of help. The most difficult part is to try and sort out the type of counselling you need. Going to the BACP website (see ref section) and looking there can help you to decide. When partners fall out and have problems couple counselling can help to sort problems out.	Counselling can be very empowering and certainly helps an individual when they are stuck. To have that listening ear can make life a lot easier. C & M

Maintaining Well Being

Some information about diet (this information is not an endorsement but different views and approaches that are available and offered by practitioners and health professionals. If in doubt always seek professional help)

In her book, The Menopause Diet, Larrain Gillespie PhD says that where menopausal women put fat on is as a result of their drop in oestrogen and progesterone. They tend to stop putting weight on hips and thighs and it is more likely fat will be stored in the stomach area. Women who are menopausal have less muscle and so less capacity to burn food so it is easy to begin to put weight on. In a survey in America weight gain was cited as the number one complaint of menopausal women.

During the change the ovaries begin to slow down production of oestrogen and progesterone, they carry on producing a hormone called androgen which can be converted to oestrogen in the fat cells. The extra fat women gain during the menopause helps produce oestrogen which can in turn alleviate some menopausal symptoms. Life style and eating habits may have to be explored and small adjustments adopted to allow for the changes caused by the menopause.

Exercise can help to build and maintain muscle mass, which will help to increase metabolic rate. If the muscle mass begins to decrease there will be less food burning cells in the body to deal with food intake.

Marilyn Glenville PhD, who wrote the New Natural Alternative to HRT, tells women in her book that the menopause is experienced differently around the world. Looking at Japanese or Chinese women they appear to have fewer symptoms of the menopause than women in the West. This is where the interest in soy products has come from as an aid to women who are experiencing menopausal problems.

There has been some negative research into soy as a supplement for the menopause. However Marilyn Glenville PhD, would suggest that soy when used as a whole food and not as a part food product there is no problem. Soy is not meant to be eaten raw or as a part product, neither is it to be eaten in excessive quantities. She would advocate that labels need to be read carefully and to avoid GM products as well as ensuring products such as soy milk are organic. In the book the Green Pharmacy J A Duke PhD suggests that women who eat a diet that contains soy products have less hot flushes and more cells in the lining of the vagina. He says that 200 grms of soy beans provide 300 mgs of phytoestrogens.

Soy is not the only food that contains Phyteostrogens and variety is the key. While it is true that soy contains a high level of Phyteostrogens, food such as legumes, aduki beans, kidney beans, garlic, seeds and grains contain good levels as well. In the book Menopause for Dummies the recommendation for eating soy is one portion per day which can be found in tofu, tempeh, soy milk and soy yoghurt, soy beans are now available in the shops. (Readers need to be aware that some people do have sensitivity to soy products)

N.B. Readers need to be aware that if there is a history of endometrioses that the phyteostrogens could start the symptoms up again. It is important to check with your GP.

Women often worry about fats; however some fats are important to help maintain hormone levels in the body. Oils in the diet are important to help skin, joints, nails, hair and depression. Essential fats also help in the absorption of calcium. The best source of essential oils for the body is via the intake of food such as vegetables, fish oils, olive oil, nut oil, and eating fish such as mackerel and salmon.

Linseed (flax) oil is good as it contains all the essential oils the body needs.

Calcium is important for bone health Miriam Stoppard in her book, Menopause, suggests the best sources of calcium comes from eating a varied diet of peas, beans, green leafy vegetables, fish, seeds, nuts, yoghurt, skimmed milk, cheese and wholemeal bread.

The uptake of vitamin D is important for ingested calcium as it helps to maintain bone density as it aids the absorption of calcium and phosphorus into the body. The main sources of vitamin D are sunlight and oily fish. (Please be sensible where sunlight is concerned as malignant melanoma is on the increase in the United Kingdom)

Fruit and vegetables are good sources of vitamins and minerals and fibre helps you to feel full as well as maintaining the vitamins and minerals the body needs.

Carbohydrates help to give energy and increase serotonin levels which assist in controlling mood and appetite. Menopausal women, according to Dr Miriam Stoppard, can have blood sugar swings that can affect their hunger levels. Women during the change may find that they are hungry sooner than they use to be. This can lead to binging especially on carbohydrate type of foods. Eating little and often can help to alleviate this problem. Ways of avoiding weight gain is by eating foods such as oats, vegetable soups and whole grain foods rather than cakes, biscuits or other high sugar and fat laden carbohydrates.

Exercise is important although the word can cause some women to flee when the word is mentioned! The best form of activity (exercise) is one that will be maintained. Many of the books that are written about the menopause talk about load bearing activities that would be included in a gym programme. It is important to start somewhere if you enjoy gardening then the green gym is a good way to increase activity, digging in the garden, raking the lawn can give a good aerobic work out activities in the garden will include some load bearing activity.

Joining a walking group, dance class, yoga or learning to play tennis or swimming are all activities that can help physical wellbeing. If you are doing something you hate there will be no enjoyment and the task will become a chore to be avoided. It is far better to do a physical activity you enjoy and gain some benefit than to do an activity you hate do it badly or give up all together.

Just to add a bit of humour "Maggie, bless her, is dyslexic and it is my job to proof read any text. At an exhibition we were attending I took the opportunity of checking the latest text for our Workshop manual. Under the exercise section Maggie had written 'Plates' and 'Swinging'! When I queried this with her she explained it was meant to be 'Pilates' and 'Swimming'!!! Well, the thought of adding Circus plate spinning on poles had us in stitches. We also tried to justify Swinging by saying it was weight bearing and a good cardio-vascular workout and toyed with the idea of including phone numbers of those willing to join in!!!! We laughed so much that the other exhibitors around us wanted to know why we were having such a good time. C

Some herbs that have been cited as helpful in the menopause

Black Cohosh – helps to increase oestrogen levels and is said to help with hot flushes - Contains licaria a natural oestrogen compound. (There are some scientific studies to back that this herb helps with hot flushes)

Chasteberry – This helps to normalise female sex hormones gives a beneficial oestrogen effect. No scientific back up research.

Red Clover can be taken in tea and is said to help with hot flushes. There have only been a few studies carried out so far.

There are some food groups that may help to balance oestrogen levels in the blood as they contain boran – 3 mg boran is said to double blood levels of oestrogen in the blood.

The highest level is found in strawberries, peaches, cabbage tomatoes and dandelion.

Other food thought to help (and they also contain phyoestrogens) are wild yams, passion flower, fennel, apple and celery stalks

Source Green Pharmacy by J A Duke PhD and the internet research

Chapter 7

Mental wellbeing

When the hormones are raging and life becomes difficult having a structure to help manage the mind can help to pull things back to reality. Trying to be rational when the physical body is making changes can be difficult, especially when in a nano second confidence disappears and anxiety and self doubt replace it.

It can be hard to recognise with all these changes going on in a woman's body that thinking may be becoming irrational and life stressful. It is easy to slip into a downward spiral and feel out of control. Hopefully if this is the case for you the following may help. You might find it useful to have a pencil handy to fill in this section.

Some women find that things change for them emotionally as they enter the menopause. It may be for example that caring for everyone was paramount and now it is not that way. It can be a difficult time and using some of the techniques below can help to keep you focused and not tumbling into everyone else's stuff and to recognise the signs and symptoms when you feel stressed or just tired!

Stress is a normal bodily reaction and as long as we can rise to the occasion when required and return to an unstressed state when things are fine. The difficulty arises when the stress becomes prolonged. This is when ill health either physically or psychologically, or a combination of both may start to kick in. When the stress response is turned on for long periods and the body does not have time to recover the immune system becomes weakened and the body become vulnerable to illness.

Identifying your Stressors and Triggers

What is a stressor/trigger? It is anything that can cause the stress response within an individual it does not necessarily have to be negative, however, usually when looking at managing stress it is the negative stressors that caused the stress response that are looked at.

Stress triggers or stressor can be activated by:-

- The environment – this can be to do with environmental space and how the individual can live within that space. These can be living space, work space; aspect such as noise, light levels, overcrowding, temperature and pollution.
- Life stress - day to day aspects of trying to live life such as travel to work, balance of home and work commitments, financial aspects, demands of family/ relationships/friendships, personal demands/expectations and life changes. Significant life change can be very stressful such as divorce, death, illness, moving house, even events such as wedding and Christmas can rate high on the stress scale.
- Work stress -related to job, role in organisation, relationships within the organisation, career development, home/work conflicts, work culture and structure, amount of control and influence over job and work practice, targets and deadlines, job skills, training.
- Personal stress- how the individual views the external world and the way that interpretation is processed internally.

Look at the list and tick the ones below that apply to you

- Feelings about yourself i.e. lack of confidence in your own skills or abilities
- Expectations too low
- Family commitments
- Children
- Spouse/partner
- Work life
- Home life

- or high
- Unrealistic expectations from self and others.
- Low self esteem/ lack of confidence
- Poor communications
- Change of environments
- Financial problems
- Relationships
- Poor health
- Too little or too much responsibility
- Time too much/too little
- Family

- Friends
- Social life

Add any that you feel are relevant to you personally

-
-
-
-
-
-

Starting to think about managing stress, it is important to recognise what our personal signs and symptoms are. Looking at the triggers and stressors that can lead to stress helps in how to develop strategies and ways to deal with the causes of stress.

Stress can contribute or be the cause of one of the following illnesses - irritable bowel syndrome, ulcers, skin problems, cardiovascular disease, migraines, high blood pressure, autoimmune diseases, depression, anxiety, substance abuse, and other mental problems.

Think about the things that cause you to become stressed. What presses your buttons? Be specific as to why they are stressful i.e. not enough time to complete my work due to other demands such as... Unhappy about unrealistic expectations others have about my ability to... I have too many things to do day to day the family/work/house...

Now fill in the box below

```


```

Learning that the contribution you may make to the stressful situation or event, by the way you behave, react to or think about the stressful situation can make it more stressful. It may be hard to recognise how we react to or think about an event may help to increase the level of stress. It is not about the event or situation itself it more about how we process within our head what is going on around us.

Internal and External Worlds- Why is it that some people seem able to cope with very stressful situations or a number of life events while others crumble at the first hurdle? Why is it that some people are able to detach and ride above very uncomfortable and difficult situations?

Why is it that some people don't fly off the handle while others throw their toys out of the pram given the same situation or event? Why is it that some individuals seem confident and self assured while others are full of anxiety and panics in the same situation?

Have a think about what things make up your values, attitudes and beliefs. These aspects are what make up your personal moral code, in relationship to yourself, others and the world around you, Sometimes this code is referred to as an individual's core beliefs.

These core beliefs drive how you think, feel and behave in relation to people in general, relationships, day to day living, and living in the world you inhabit? This exercise enables you to think about the constituents that go to make up your core beliefs

- What are my attitudes in relationship to myself, others and the world around me?

- What are my values in relationship to myself, others and the world around me?

- What are my beliefs in relationship to myself, others and the world around me?

ABC Model

You are now building up a picture of what you are about and the things that are important to you. Go back to your list of beliefs, attitudes and values and think about how these things may affect how you live your day to day life. Where might it cause you stress or how might it affect your behaviour or build up emotions such as resentment, anger, anxiety, jealousy, frustration, rejection or powerlessness?

When we interact with the outside world or go about our daily life events happen and we find we may become angry, frustrated, anxious or any number of different emotions. Sometimes we behave in ways that don't help the situation we may find ourselves in, we may shut off, withdraw, or say things that we don't mean.

It is often easy to blame a situation on other people, an institution or the world for the strong emotions we feel or our behaviour. It is not as simple as saying the reason I am angry is because everything has gone wrong today and it is all ....fault. We often externalise what is happening internally and the way it is processed via the core beliefs filter.

When an situation/ event occurs there is a process that happens. Most people think that the event A (activating event) causes the emotion, behaviour, resultant at C (the consequences)

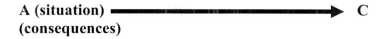

A (situation) ➤ **C**
(consequences)

I am late due to the traffic   *I am angry,*

I drive like a maniac

There is another dimension that comes into play which is our belief system and this belief or demand will drive how we react resulting in consequences.

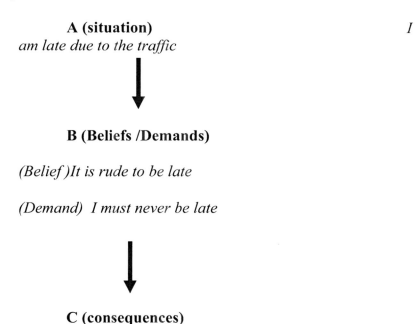

A (situation)   *I*
am late due to the traffic

B (Beliefs /Demands)

(Belief)It is rude to be late

(Demand) I must never be late

C (consequences)

I am angry, I drive like a lunatic

The result of the demand and or belief is the consequence of driving badly and the consequence of that behaviour.

66

Think about a few situations that have occurred for you over the last few days or week. What were the beliefs or demands you had about the event and what were the consequences?

Now look at the situation and see if your responses were healthy or unhealthy, think about how each aspect can affect you physically and mentally.

Aspect	Response	Healthy	Unhealthy
Thoughts			
Behaviour			
Emotions			
Bodily responses			

What conclusion have you come to?

-
-
-
-
-

You are beginning to build up a profile of how you react to events and situations on a daily basis and whether the responses are healthy or unhealthy. Hopefully you are beginning to understand that how you process the world internally has an effect both internally and externally. If the response is healthy no damage is done and you have wellbeing. However if the responses are unhealthy this is where the problems begin to arise.

Internal Thoughts and External Effects

The way we process our thoughts in our heads can produce emotions, physical symptoms and behaviour that could potentially be harmful to our bodies if our thinking processes are irrational or unhealthy.

When our internal thinking processes are realistic, rational and healthy this will lead to balance, calm and well being. This will mean that the thinking is rational and keeping things in perspective. Emotions will be healthy and behaviour constructive and helpful. Thinking this way keeps demands and expectations realistic, self worth high, maintains motivation, goal setting is realistic and achievable, maintains good time and self management, communication and relationship are good.

If on the other hand our internal thinking processes are irrational, unrealistic and unhealthy this will lead to thinking that lacks perspective and clarity such as jumping to conclusions, demands and expectations are unrealistic. Emotions will be unhealthy and behaviour destructive and unhelpful. Unrealistic thinking leads to stress, anxiety, anger, panic, depression, and addictive behaviour. Self worth plummets, time and self management become chaotic, relationships and communications suffer, motivation falls, goal are unrealistic,

Our thought processes affect the way we think feel and behave in the External world

External World

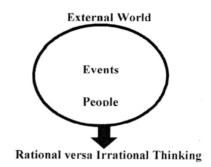

Events

People

Rational versa Irrational Thinking

Internal world

Negative option   Positive option

Thoughts -
Irrational/unrealistic

Thoughts- rational
/realistic

Emotions –unhealthy

Emotions-healthy

Behaviour –destructive

Behaviour –constructive

Results in Stress, anxiety,
anger, depression,
unrealistic demands
expectations, lack of
confidence

Results in calm, realistic
demands and
expectations, Confidence

Thinking Errors

When we do not think rationally we produce thinking errors, it helps to recognise the type of errors we have when we start to process information within our brain. The list below gives eight types of errors which can help you to learn to recognise the type of mistakes individuals can make in thinking. Helping to understand how to rectify errors, problem solving or dispute unrealistic thinking helps to develop a brain that will help you to gain wellbeing.

Read the list and see if you recognise any errors in your thinking.

Error 1 <u>Catastrophization</u>

This where a small negative event is blown up into a disaster.

'I spilt my drink all over the table and now my friend will not invite me back ever again'.

Change thinking –Use factual descriptions, and look for the evidence for statements that say how terrible things are. Weigh up the evidence and look at how realistic thoughts are.

Error 2 <u>Demandingness/perfectionism</u>

Having inflexible demands/ expectations about self the world and other people.

'I must perform well otherwise I am a failure'

'they should not do that job that way -what a waste of time'

Change thinking –Be aware of thoughts that demand that the world runs according to personal rules and that people have to behave as you demand they do. Try to avoid using words like must, should, got to - try using alternatives such as rather, wish and prefer. Have your own beliefs but don't demand that others have the same ones as you, be flexible. E.g. You would prefer everyone liked you, or you would rather you did your job well.

Error 3 <u>Discounting the positive</u>

This is where positive events are translated into a negative event.

'When I get a good appraisal my manager doesn't really mean it because I don't deserve it'

Change thinking –Think of the situation using factual information only; try to reframe the negative thoughts with more realistic ones. It is important to accept when you have done something well by praising yourself for a good job done instead of always finding fault.

Error 4 <u>Fortune telling</u>

Being a psychic looking into the future predicting what will happen, which is usually negative.

'I was late this morning due to an accident, so the rest of the day will be awful'

Change thinking- The key is to be as open minded as possible. Try to avoid making judgments about what is going to happen. You don't know what is going to occur until it actually happens. Take a few risks; test out your predictions; was the rest of the day awful? Just because things have happened in the past it does not follow it will happen again. Could try to use a scale to look at the possibility of something happening again e.g. somewhere between 0-100% ask yourself why you have given the rating you have and how realistic it is.

Error 5 <u>Mind-reading</u>

Assuming other people have negative thoughts/words /views about you.

'I'm know my colleagues think I am not pulling my weight'

Change thinking- Unless some one tells you how they are thinking you don't know what is in their heads. Generate alternatives. Someone may behave or respond as they have for reasons you may not have considered.

Error 6 <u>Overgeneralisation/Exaggeration-</u>

This is drawing wide conclusions from one or two small events/incidents

'Everyone hates me I was silly to lose my temper now no one will ever talk to me again'

Change thinking- Avoid globalizing events or situations, rather put events into perspectives. Think how someone else might view the situation. Be specific, keep to the facts you know. Avoid using words such as always, never, everyone, the whole world

Error7 *<u>Worth Rating</u>*

This is where an individual rates their worth by performance, results, people's opinions, abilities and/or possessions.

'Since my partner left I am nothing , I am no one without a partner'

Change thinking - Avoid valuing things you do against wealth, position or status. Base your self -worth on something that doesn't change. Challenge negative thoughts and replace them with the truth. Notice when you act in inferior/ unworthy ways and try and find something that is positive or good about you i.e. I have a good sense of humour. I was able to do that part well. The value of self-worth is having confidence in who you are without conforming to the expectations of other people.

Error 8 **All or nothing thinking**

This is where thinking goes from one extreme to another where things are either great or awful with no in between.

'Now I have eaten a chocolate I have failed on my diet I might as well eat the whole box'

Change thinking- Check out how realistic your thinking is; do reality checks. Imagine you could score the reality in your thinking. If you are realistic how bad it is? You can make a few slips and still obtain the goal i.e. eat a few chocolates and still lose weight.

When thinking is chaotic, unrealistic and demanding and when events, relationships and communications become distorted this is when people lose control and feel they have no choice. The people who are in control and driving their own thinking and emotions are the ones who don't lose the plot and keep control in their lives. They are the ones who can jump over the hurdles of life.

There are other types of thinking errors and in the index you will find books on Cognitive Behavioural Therapy which will give you more types of errors if you are interested

Disputing Thoughts

You may need a process to help you dispute irrational thoughts. Sometimes you may need a little help to get your brain into a more rational mode. If you are feeling anxious, stressed, and angry or you could have a headache, irritable bowel or have your heart racing. Sometimes you can feel yourself just becoming hot and bothered and don't know why.

Use one of the examples you have used in a previous exercise and see if you can reframe the situation by following the process below.

1. What evidence is there about the thought?
    - Evidence to support thought
    - Evidence against the thought

2. What alternative views/thoughts
    - How would someone else view it (i.e. a best friend)?
    - How might you have viewed it in the past?

3. What might be the result or consequence of continuing to think in this way?
    - Is it helpful?
    - Will it help to get what is wanted?
    - How might it hinder?
    - What are the emotional/physical/ behavioural/interpersonal consequences?

4. What may have caused distorted or unrealistic thinking

Catastrophization	
Demandingness/Perfectionism	
Disqualifying the Positives	
Fortune Telling	
Mind Reading	

Overgeneralisation/Exaggeration	
Worth Rating	
All or nothing thinking	

5. What action can be taken?
   - ➢ What can be altered?
   - ➢ What is working?
   - ➢ What can't be altered?

6. Where does that leave me now?

7. How can I reframe my thinking to be more realistic?

(Adapted from E- book Stress Being to Wellbeing © pacetherapy - www.pacetherapy.co.uk)

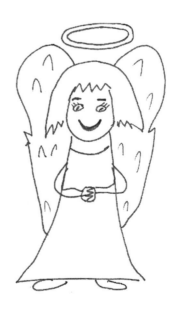

End note

Some women may have had years of managing the family, the household and often extended families as well. It is likely that a woman is also working either full or part-time on top of everything else. It is so easy to lose sight of "me". Gaining back "me" space is not always easy, especially when it has been the lesser of two evils just to say yes. Trying to get a perspective of what is important for "me" for where I am here and now, does require some thought and this is why some women become so down and emotional because things are changing and it is hard to cope as they have done so in the past.

At this time it can be hard to make decisions especially if you are struggling with tiredness, hot flushes and raging emotions. Trying to understand what is important as well as establishing the things that can be let go is not always easy. I certainly had to step back at times and tell myself it was ok to give myself a little slack and that there was only 24 hrs in the day. When I was feeling worn out some things had to go or just wait. However when I was feeling down I had to use the thinking errors to keep things in perspective. Not easy when some of those around me expected me to create miracles and be super woman. Taking care of me was important. When I was tearful or getting angry it was my signs that I needed time out or a little space.

For some women being more assertive and learning to say no is important. One of the ways to manage the symptoms of the menopause is to recognise our own needs and wants. When women are tired and trying to deal with life and every day needs and wants from friends and relatives learning to say no can be so helpful. If it is difficult for you to say no then taking an assertive course may be beneficial. In the courses I teach on Assertiveness it is usually the biggest problem for course participants to say no, I ask about them and where are they in the picture it certainly makes them start to think as they begin to see that they are important as well. When you say yes when you really mean no you become more tired and life becomes more difficult so saying no does make life easier in the long run. Maggie

I have found it quite hard at times to know where my thoughts are coming from and this has made me very wary about making important decisions. Is it the hormones talking or me? Which is why I feel it is important to understand what has been written in this section especially the thinking errors.

If I'm angry, anxious or not very confident on a particular day I wonder if my feelings or emotions are down to a hormone surge. It is so easy to be swept away by an emotion which is why I tend not to make life changing decision until I know I am back in control. Chris

Even though   *By Maggie Stanley*

Even though I look in the mirror
And see a woman I don't recognise
I am still me

Even though my hormones rage
And I appear muddled and forgetful
I am still me

Even though my body's changing
And mind is misbehaving
I am still me

Even though my life is not as before
Things ending, things beginning
I am still me

Even though the woman I was

Is fading, my uniqueness is unfolding
I am still me

Even though I'm in a chrysalis
I am breaking free
To soar to fly
To be uniquely me

Chapter 8

Some useful tips and Information

Using Emotional Freedom Technique

I have found EFT to be very beneficial in lots of circumstances but the one occasion that relates just on menopause happened last year when with a group of friends.

We had gone away for a joint birthday celebration. We were all hitting 50 that year and felt it was something to celebrate as well as our long friendship. Going for breakfast in the large dining room one morning I noticed one of my friends turning beetroot red and grabbing the menu to fan herself. We jokingly refer to 'Tropical Moments' and I asked her if she was having one? She was mortified because it had taken her by surprise. I then offered to help her by doing some EFT (Emotional Freedom Technique).

I asked her first of all what it was that was upsetting her, the hot flush, feeling embarrassed etc? She said it was the embarrassment. I then asked her on a scale of 1-10 how bad that feeling was? She said

10! I then tapped her hand and said "Even though I am SO embarrassed I'm OK". The great thing about EFT is that you don't actually have to believe what you are saying because it is NOT an affirmation.

I then continued to tap at the start of her brow saying "I know I'm in public" side of her eye "everyone is watching me" under her nose "God only knows what they are thinking of me", under her bottom lip "I'm really showing myself up", 'Tarzan' point" I feel so miserable", bra line under arm "why is my body letting me down?". I finished with her repeating after me again "Even though I am SO embarrassed I'm Ok". I asked her to take a deep breath and sip some water. I then asked her on 1-10 scale how she was feeling now. She said "5"! We had one more go but on the bra line this time I put in "I'm never going to see these people again so what's the problem?" She laughed at this and after her 'score' was 2. In just 3 minutes her flush had gone from full-on and uncomfortable to gone! She was amazed and I was so glad that I was able to help her out.

EFT for Menopause, Hot flushes and Chills

Typically, menopausal symptoms such as hot flushes and chills last anywhere from a few months to a few years. Depending on their severity, they can affect sleep, relationships, job performance and a long list of important life functions.

For those of us who do not want to go down the route of HRT then EFT could be the answer.

I have already mentioned elsewhere in this book my success with my friend on using EFT for her hot flush so thought I would explain a bit more on how to use it for yourselves.

It's very important to have the 'set-up' phrase correct at the beginning. Remember, it is NOT an affirmation and you don't have to actually believe in it for this to work!

Also, remember to take a 'score' of the intensity of how you're feeling BEFORE you start. On a scale of 1-10 (10 worst you can feel, 1-everything ok)

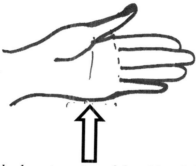

(Tapping firmly on the karate point of the side of the hand firmly while repeating this out loud three times)

"Even though I suffer from these menopausal symptoms, they are a part of the natural ageing process, and I'm OK"

I then eventually added the following to each tapping spot....

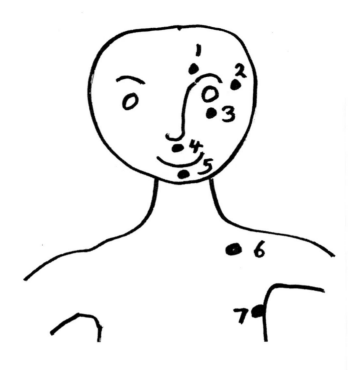

"and I want these symptoms to stop now"

I then move to more specifics:

"Even though I have these _____ (i.e. horrible, annoying, exhausting, tiring, embarrassing, etc.) hot flushes, I'm ok"

"Even though I am still having some_____ hot flushes I understand this is normal, and I want them to STOP now, I'm ok"

Continue tapping and adding "remaining" and "residual" to the reminder phrases as appropriate. You may find while tapping on one aspect you automatically come out with something different, which sometimes happens. Focus on that until you bring down the intensity of the emotion.

"Even though I am suffering from these____ *(i.e. horrible, annoying, exhausting, tiring, embarrassing, etc.)* ' night sweats' I'm ok because this is a normal phase of life and I just want them to STOP now.

Hopefully you will find the symptoms lessening. If you find it too difficult to concentrate on doing the tapping etc yourself then book to see a qualified EFT Practitioner for at least one session so that you can be shown how to do it correctly. Preferably find someone who belongs to an association with Codes of Conduct and Ethics.

A Barbie we can relate to

Lou Ann Thomas is a freelance writer from Jefferson County who wrote an article in 2000 for the Topeks Capital-Journal called "Barbie should have reflected the changing Baby Boomers".

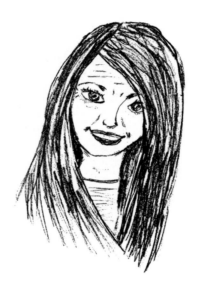

The article suggested that Mattel should have produced a Barbie to match every stage of the Baby Boomers life. The theme of her piece has inspired many to quote it in forums and website across the internet. Such Barbie's are hot flush Barbie, bifocal Barbie, facial hair Barbie, mid life crisis Barbie, divorce Barbie who comes with Ken's car and house the list is very funny and worth a look at.

The link to the article is as follows - http://findarticles.com/p/articles/mi_qn4179/is_20000601/ai_n117482 50

The link to A Barbie we can relate to is as follows –

Chapter 9

Some book websites and help lines that may be useful

We would not have been able to write some aspects of this book without being able to research information from some of the books and websites we have mentioned below.

Books about the menopause –There are a number of books that deal with the subject some are more medical in approach and some are more self help like diet and remedies. Some of these we have found helpful and have assisted in the writing of this book.

Menopause and the mind By Claire Warga PhD Touchstone press ISBN 0-684 85479 1

Menopause for Dummies by Brewer, Jones and Eichenwald Pub John Wiley and Sons IBSN 978 0 470 06100-8

Menopause by Dr Miriam Stoppard Pub Dorling Kindersley ISBN 0-7513 0082 9

Hormone Replacement Therapy By Rosemary Nicol Pub Vermillion ISBN 0-09 177666-x

The New Natural Alternatives to HRT by M Glenville PhD pub Kyle Cathie Ltd ISBN 1-85626-582-x

The Menopause Diet By Larrian Gillespie Pub Healthier Life ISBN 0-96771317-7-1

After the Change by Kathleen Griffin pub vermilion

ISBN 0-09-181345-3

Women's Bodies Women's Wisdom by Dr Christiane Northrup pub piatkus ISBN0-7499-1925-6

Books on different subjects that may be of help These books range from complimentary approaches to help with the more emotional side of life.

The Green Pharmacy By J A Duke PhD Pub Rodale - give good information on how diet can help with some of the symptoms of the menopause.

The Fragrant Pharmacy By V A Worwood pub Bantom Books ISBN 0-533 40397-4 Good book to read up about different aromatherapy oils and how they may help symptoms.

Bach Flower Therapy by Mechthild Scheffer Pub Thorsons ISBN 0-7225 1121-3 Gives more information about how these flower essences can help with the emotional side of life.

The Complete Homeopathy Handbook by Miranda Castro Pub Macmillion ISBN 0-33-55581-3 – Good reference book to look at how homeopathy can help with symptoms.

Cognitive Behavioural Therapy for Dummies Pub Wilson Branch ISBN 0-470-01838-0 Very readable and helpful book for people struggling with thinking errors a simple no nonsense approach.

The Feeling Good Handbook by DD Burns MD Pub Plume Books ISBN 0-452 26174-0 - More in depth book about handling emotions and behaviour good sections but quite a big book.

Change Your Thinking by Dr S Edelman Pub Vermillion ISBN 0-09190 695-4

Think Your Way to Happiness By Dryden And Gordon Pub Sheldon Press ISBN 0-85969 603-0 This book is a little book on challenging emotions and behaviour not as simple and "how to " as the CBT for dummies

Teach Yourself to Meditate by Eric Harrision Pub Piatkus ISBN 0-749 1328-2 well written book and the author helps the individual to realise they can learn to meditate.

Why Men Don't Listen And Women Can't Read Maps by A And B Pease Pub P.T.I IBSN 0-6463 4907 4 This book is great written by a male and female psychologist who are married it helps the reader to understand the differences between male and female.

Web sites and Contact Details for help lines and organisations

Directly for the menopause

www.menopausematters.co.uk Dumfries based Helpline (DGRI) - 01387 241121Thursday mornings 9am to 12 noon (Gives advice / information about menopause, HRT, natural alternatives, and osteoporosis).

British Menopause Society www.the-bms.org Women's Health concern Ltd.10 Storey's Gate, Westminster, London. SW1P 3AY Nurse counselling service: 0845 123 2319 www.womens-health-concern.org

The GP Training website has a whole range of pages with very useful information. Go to the section for patients and just put in the topic in the search box and information will come up. Link – www.gp-training.net or the try the links below

The Menopause self help guide is brilliant it takes each aspect of the menopause give advice on diet, exercise, remedies and herbs. Link -

www.gp training.net/pal/therapy/hrtselfhelp.htm

Vaginal dryness – good advice about how to cope with and products to help with problem-link www.gp-training.net/pal/gynaecology/vaginal_dryness.htm

Pelvic floor exercises for stress incontinence this section is very good about bladder advice and gives some exercises to help with incontinence. Link-www.gp-training.net/pal/gynaecology/pelvicfloorexcercises.htm

Menopausal Symptoms and CAM a very good site for information on Phytoestrogens and botanical (plant extract) and complimentary approaches.   Link http://nccam.nih.gov/health/menopauseandcam/

Is HRT safe? Written by Dr Dan Rutherford, GP a good article to look at if you are unsure about taking HRT Link - www.netdoctor.co.uk/womenshealth/facts/hrt.htm

NHS Direct for information about the menopause and HRT Link - http://cks.library.nhs.uk/menopause#-278118

The National Osteoporosis Society Camerton, Bath. BA2 0PS Telephone – 0176 147 1771 (office) 0845 450 0230 (helpline) Fax 0176 147 1104 Website - www.nos.org.uk

Alliance pharmacy To help you to decide if you need to check up about the medication you are taking.
www.alliancepharmacy.co.uk/index.php?link=ourservices&sublink=services&subsublink=medicinescheckup

Daisy Network registered charity for women suffering premature menopause PO Box 392, High Wycombe, Bucks. HP15 7SH
www.daisynetwork.org.uk

Remedies for Menopausal Symptoms
www.project-aware.org/Managing/Alt/index_remedies.shtml -

Other useful websites and helplines

Mind Information Line: 08457 660 163 if you live elsewhere (9.15am-4.45pm Mon, Wed & Thur) www.mind.org.uk

Hidden Hurt – domestic violence www.hiddenhurt.co.uk/

Bullying help line: Andrea Adams Trust 01273 704900

Carers- Government information for Carers
www.carers.gov.uk/index.htm

Crossroads - Caring for Carers www.crossroads.org.uk/
01788-573653

Alzheimer's Society www.alzheimers.org.uk/ Helpline: 0845 300 0336 (8.30am-6.30pm Mon-Fri)

NHS Stop Smoking www.givingupsmoking.co.uk NHS Smoking Helpline: 0800 169 0 169 freecall

British Assoc Counselling and Psychotherapy www.bacp.co.uk 08704435252

Products

Chillow Pillow Available from http://www.gizoo.co.uk **£24.95**

Coolsleepwear.co.uk is a new website selling the Wildbleu™ brand of nightwear, which uses wicking technology to promote restful sleep. The range is available online at www.coolsleepwear.co.uk.

Chapter 10

Menopause Survey

When Chris and I first started talking about running courses for women on the menopause we decided it would be a good idea to talk to women and ask about their experience. We devised a survey, not an academic one, to try and establish what women wanted, which aspects of this life experience they found difficult, and what was helping or had helped them.

Chris and I have both come across women in the change who were finding life difficult emotionally so we decided to include a section on mental well being.

The anecdotal information women gave us was a fascinating insight into the different way women experience this time of life. There were women who sailed through gracefully with very few problems and on the other side there were women who were having or had a very rough time.

Women did seem to feel that there was little information about the change and that the menopause was seen as a medical problem, not as a stage in life such as puberty.

During the time that the surveys were conducted we certainly had some laughs with women about memory lapses, urine leeks and hot flushes. We also heard some sad stories of women let down by being ill informed or not being listened to.

I think that Chris and I were humbled by the fact that a short conversation with a woman about the menopause could create such a change. We found they felt empowered less emotionally down as they understood what was happening to them. On the relationship side to realise that the intimate aspects of their lives did not have to end and that there were things that could be done.

At the time of writing the survey has been completed by 50 women. The analysis of the survey is showing up some interesting information. (If any one would like the full results please contact (maggie@paceuk.com).

60% of responders said that hot flushes were the most difficult symptom to deal with. Second at 50% was disturbed sleep, weight gain and memory lapses/loss.

Nearly 40% of women stated that they were having disturbed sleep nightly and 33% having to deal with daily memory lapses and forgetfulness.

Over 45% said they would like information about how complementary and alternative treatments could help with the menopause.

The concerns and fears that most women had were to do with hot flushes/ night sweats and mood swings.
87% of women who answered the survey are not taking Hormone Replacement Therapy and 81% had never taken the treatment.

The women who responded to the section on personal recommendations to help with the menopause nearly 41% responders advocated herbal treatments and supplements and nearly 26% recommended complimentary therapies.

This was an interesting exercise and we are grateful to the ladies who completed the survey. Not only did they give us important information they also gave us an opportunity to learn and widen our experience, so a big thank you to all of you.

Biogs

Maggie and Chris met in 1996 on a Reiki course in Margate, Kent. There was an instant connection and the course tutor threatened to separate them on several occasions. They came together to form Stress Busting Angels a few years ago their interest complimentary therapies and the different approaches make them an interesting working partnership. They bring their unique warmth, fun and humour to workshops and therapy.

Details and information about menopause courses can be found on their website www.stressbustingangels.co.uk

Maggie originally trained as a hypnotherapist and soon became interested in stress and behaviour change. She studied Stress Management which led her to train in other therapies such as Reiki healing Indian Head massage and EFT.

Maggie also runs workshops and develops training packages. She is a co director of Stress Busting Angels with Chris Guyon.

Maggie worked for the NHS for a number of years as a Cardiac technician and most recently as a specialist Stop Smoking Advisor. She taught counselling skills and assertiveness in adult education for a number of years. Maggie's keen interest in behaviour change led her on to becoming involved with The University of West England co writing the behaviour change module for the NHS health Trainers course. Maggie also works as a freelance trainer for South Gloucester PCT, delivering psyco/ social skill to patients.   Maggie is a volunteer for Somerset Cancer Care.

Chris Guyon was drawn to Reiki eleven years ago and over a period of five years worked her way through each level and finally became a Reiki Master. Although she worked in the NHS for over thirty years in different areas she finally gave up the 'day job' to concentrate on her Reiki Practice and teaching Reiki to students who wished to access this energy for their own well-being and for others. As well as running her practice she was part of a team of Complementary Therapists who were employed by her local Council to go into the Civic Offices to de-stress staff in the workplace. This proved to be very popular with the staff! Chris also offered her services to the local Primary Care Trust and would go into Health Centres and Clinics during staff lunch hours to give de-stressing sessions. She also gives voluntary Reiki sessions at her local Women's Refuge.

Three years ago Chris trained as an EFT Practitioner. After knowing Maggie for eleven years she decided it was time to pool their knowledge and experiences and Stress Busting Angels was born!

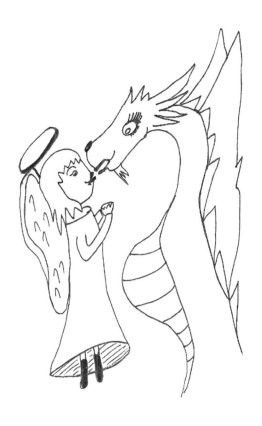

Lightning Source UK Ltd.
Milton Keynes UK
26 April 2010

153351UK00002B/189/P